WELLNESS WAVELENGHTS

Self care For Busy Professionals

More than 400 Tips For Healthy Lifestyle

Hajra Begum

Preface

Introduction In today's busy world, maintaining good health can often be a difficult task. The bombardment of information, fads, and conflicting advice can make it difficult to know where to start or who to trust. This guide is designed to serve as a beacon of trustworthy information, providing practical advice, evidence-based strategies, and expert tips to help you improve your physical, mental, and emotional health. Whether you're starting a new health journey or looking to improve your current habits, this guide will give you the tools you need to make informed decisions and achieve your health goals. We believe that health is more than the absence of disease, but a complete state of physical, mental, and social well-being.

By taking a holistic approach to health, focusing on nutrition, exercise, sleep, stress management, and mindfulness, you can build a strong foundation for a healthy, fulfilling life. Remember, small changes can bring big results.

Begin your journey to better health with an open mind and a willingness to prioritize your health. Health is your most valuable asset, and by investing in yourself, you will lay the foundation for a happier, stronger, and more resilient future. We hope that this guide will be a valuable companion on your health journey. May it inspire, empower, and guide you toward a life of strength and balance. Wishing you good health!

Hajra Begum

Table Of Contents

Table
Of Contents

Table
Of Contents

Hair

Hair is a thread-like natural substance that emerges from tiny pockets in the skin of animals, humans included. Mainly made up of a substance known as keratin, hair has multiple roles, such as shielding, keeping warm, and sensing. It is crucial in shaping our social and cultural identities, affecting trends and how we express ourselves. The characteristics of hair, like its feel, hue, and length, are determined by our genes and the surroundings. More than just a biological element, hair holds great cultural importance, often representing attractiveness, social standing, and personal uniqueness.

Hair issues can come from many things like genes, how you live, what you eat, and your surroundings. Here are some common problems:

1. Hair Loss (Alopecia): This can happen for different reasons like genes, hormones, stress, health issues, or certain drugs.

2. Dandruff: This is when your scalp flakes. It can be from dry skin, bad reactions to hair products, fungal infections, or other skin problems.

3. Dry and Damaged Hair: This is from too much styling, too much heat, harsh products, the environment, or not taking good care of your hair.

4. Split Ends: These happen when your hair splits or frays because of damage.

5. Grey Hair: This is normal as you age because of less melanin. But, you might start grey earlier if you have certain genes, are stressed, or have a bad lifestyle.

With the help of below tips we combat many hair problems:

1.Nutrition:
  - Incorporate a well-balanced diet filled with essential vitamins, minerals, and proteins.

  - Add foods such as seafood, nuts, fruits, vegetables, and whole grains to your meals.

2. Hydration:
  - Stay hydrated by drinking enough water daily to ensure your hair remains moisturized from within.

3. Minimize Heat Styling:
  - Reduce the frequency of using heat tools like straighteners and curling irons to avoid damage.

4. Let It Dry Naturally:
  - Whenever feasible, allow your hair to dry naturally instead of using a blow dryer.

5. Regular Trims:
  - Schedule regular haircuts every 6-8 weeks to prevent split ends and hair breakage.

6. Gentle Detangling:
  - Use a wide-tooth comb to gently remove tangles, minimizing the risk of hair breakage.

7. Sun Protection:
   - Wear a hat or apply hair products with UV protection when you're out in the sun.

8. Silk or Satin Pillowcase:
   - Opt for a silk or satin pillowcase to reduce friction and prevent hair breakage during sleep.

9. Loose Hairstyles:
   - Choose hairstyles that are not too tight, like ponytails or braids, to avoid pulling and damage.

10. Weekly Deep Conditioning:
   - Treat your hair to a deep conditioning treatment once a week to keep it nourished and hydrated.

11. Select the Right Hair Care Products:
   - Pick shampoos and conditioners that are appropriate for your hair type and specific needs.

12. Scalp Massage:
   - Massaging your scalp can enhance blood flow and stimulate hair growth.

13. Swimming Protection:
   - Wear a swim cap or rinse your hair thoroughly after swimming to eliminate chlorine or salt water.

14. Moderate Hair Washing:
   - Aim to wash your hair 2-3 times a week to avoid stripping it of its natural oils.

15. Chlorine Defense:
  - Wet your hair with clean water before swimming to lessen the impact of chlorine.

16. Occasional Clarifying Shampoo:
  - Use a clarifying shampoo occasionally to remove any product buildup.

17. Use sulfate-free shampoos: Sulfates can strip your hair of its natural oils, so choose sulfate-free shampoos.

18. Avoid Overwashing: Washing your hair too often can strip it of its natural oils. Aim for 2-3 washes per week.

19. Rinse with Cold Water: Finish your shower with cold water to seal the hair and add shine.

20. Deep Conditioning Routine: Use a deep conditioning treatment once a week to nourish and soften your hair.

21. Avoid hair accessories: Opt for hair accessories that do not drag or pull on your hair.

22. Manage stress: Chronic stress can contribute to hair loss, so practice ways to reduce stress.

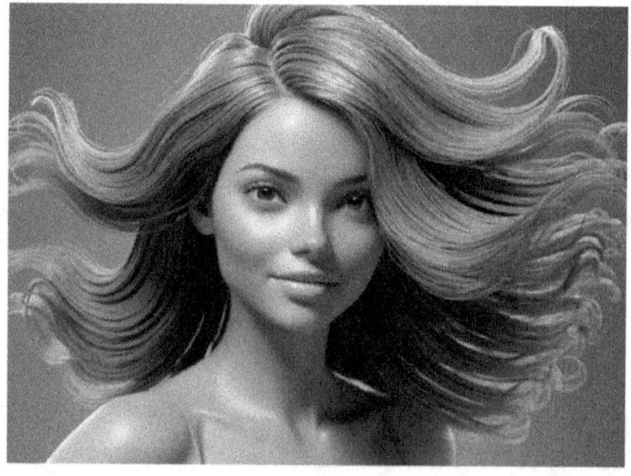

Eyes

The eyes are vital organs that play a crucial role in our daily lives and overall well-being.

Having good vision and vision is important for overall health.

Below are some tips to help you care for your eyes and protect your vision:

1. Get regular eye exams to detect problems early.

2. Eat a well-balanced diet rich in fruits, vegetables, and omega-3 fatty acids.

3. Protect your eyes from harmful UV rays by wearing sunglasses when outdoors.

4. Take frequent breaks from the screen to prevent eye strain.

5. Practice good hygiene to prevent eye infections.

6. Use good lighting when reading or working.

7. Drink plenty of water to keep your eyes healthy.

8. Maintain a healthy weight to reduce the risk of eye diseases.

9. Exercise regularly for blood pressure and eye health.

10. Avoid smoking to prevent eye diseases such as macular degeneration.

11. Use eye protection for chronic conditions such as diabetes and high blood pressure to protect your eyes.

12. Wear safety glasses during sports or activities that endanger your eyes.

13. Follow the 20-20-20 rule: every 20 minutes, take a 20-second break and look at an object 20 meters away.

14. Always keep your eyes open and bright.

15. Practice posture to reduce neck and eyes.

16. If your eyes are dry, use artificial tears or eye cream.

17. Quit or avoid alcohol to protect your eyes.

18. Control blue light exposure by using digital devices with filters or blue-blocking glasses.

19. Get good sleep so your eyes can rest and refresh.

20. Limit sugar intake to reduce the risk of eye damage.

21. Take advantage of stress to prevent eye strain and headaches.

22. Practice proper hygiene to prevent eye infection.

.23. Wash your hands before touching your eyes to prevent the spread of germs.

24. Make sure your work area is economical to reduce glare.

25. Learn your family history of eye diseases and problems.

26. Wear eye protection as prescribed to help you see better.

27. Continue to report potential eye side effects from medications you take.

28. Use an anti-glare screen on your computer to reduce glare.

29. Stay active and maintain a healthy lifestyle to support the overall health of your eyes.

30. Practice good eating habits, such as eating foods rich in vitamin A.

Dry eye,Itching and burning in eyes, conjunctivitis are easily prevent by following above tips properly.

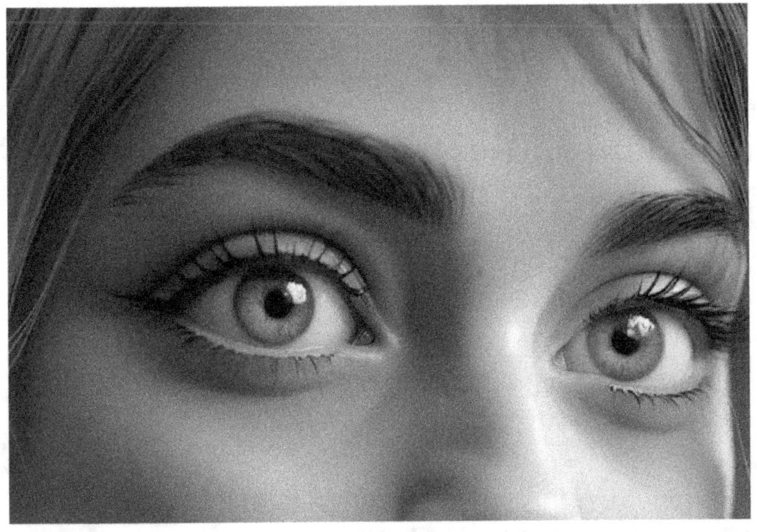

Lips

Lips are key in both talking and showing feelings. They help in speaking by making it easier to form words and sounds. Outside of talking, lips are important for showing emotions like joy, sorrow, and astonishment through gentle movements.

Moreover, lips protect the mouth and teeth from outside things. They are also delicate, filled with nerves that improve our sense of touch and taste. In addition, nice lips make a face look better, affecting how others see beauty and appeal. Therefore, the importance of lips goes beyond just how they look, affecting how we communicate, our health, and how we interact with others.

Taking care of your lips is important for your overall health and maintaining a healthy smile.

Below are some tips for healthy lips:

1. Stay hydrated: Drink plenty of water to keep your lips moist.

2. Use lip balm: Use lip balm with SPF to protect your lips from the sun.

3. Avoid licking your lips: Saliva can dry out your lips, so avoid licking them too much.

4. Gentle care: Use a mild lip scrub to remove dead skin cells and keep your lips healthy.

5. Use before bed: Apply a thick layer of lip balm before bed to moisturize your lips throughout the night.

6. Use natural oils: Coconut oil, almond oil or jojoba oil can help keep your lips soft and moisturized.

7. Do not bite your lips: Avoid biting or picking your lips; this can cause irritation and dryness.

8. Protect yourself from the cold: Wear a scarf or mask to protect your lips in cold weather.

9. Avoid harsh products: Choose lip balms and lipsticks with natural ingredients to prevent irritation.

10. Healthy diet: Eat a diet rich in vitamins and minerals to support healthy skin, including your lips.

11. Avoid smoking: Smoking can dry out your lips and cause them to become discolored, so avoid having beautiful lips.

12. Watch Out for Allergens: Some lip products can contain allergens that can irritate your lips, so be careful about what you use.

13. Use a humidifier: Place a humidifier in your room to prevent the air from drying out.

14. Stay active: Regular exercise can improve blood circulation, which can benefit your lips.

15. Remove Makeup Before Bed: Make sure to remove all lipstick and lip products before going to bed.

16. Protect Your Lips From Harsh Weather: Protect your lips from harsh weather conditions such as wind and sun.

17. Be Gentle When Removing Flakes: If your lips are chapped, gently scrub or use a wet washcloth to remove the dead skin

18. Take care of your teeth: Some toothpastes can irritate your teeth, so opt for healthy milks.

19. Avoid Dry Air: If you live in a dry environment, take special precautions to keep your lips dry.

Some below problems are easily prevent by following above tips properly

1. Chapped Lips: Dry, flaky, or cracked lips can occur due to factors like cold weather, dehydration, excessive licking, or certain medications.

2. Sunburned Lips: Prolonged sun exposure without protection can cause sunburn on the lips, leading to pain, redness, and possible blistering.

3. Infections: Bacterial or fungal infections can occur on the lips, causing symptoms like redness, swelling, pain, and sometimes draining sores.

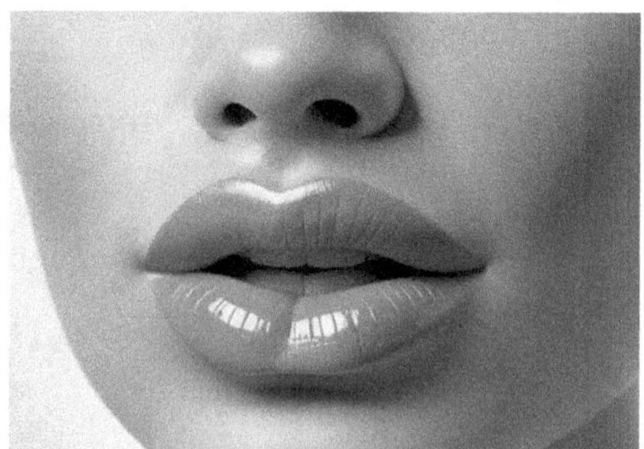

Skin

As the body's largest organ, the skin protects us from the elements, regulates physiological processes, and contributes to our overall health and well-being. Maintaining the health and function of the skin requires proper hygiene, nutrition, and sun protection.

Good skin care involves a combination of good skin care routines, a healthy lifestyle and some conscious habits.

Below are some tips to help you get and maintain healthy skin:

1. Cleanse twice a day: Use a mild cleanser in the morning and evening to remove dIrt and oil.

2. Daily use: Moisturize your skin with adequate moisture.

3. Exfoliate weekly: Remove dead skin cells with a gentle exfoliant.

4. Wear sunscreen: Protect your skin from harmful UV rays by wearing sunscreen every day.

5. Use a serum: Use a serum developed for specific skin concerns.

6. Use a face mask: Apply a face mask to your skin once or twice a week.

7. Avoid touching your face: Avoid unnecessary contact with your face to prevent bacterial infections.

8. Avoid hot showers: Hot water can strip your skin of its natural oils.

9.Swap regular pillows: Dirty pillows can cause acne.

10 Use a moisturizer: This can help your skin, especially in dry weather.

11. Do a patch test: Test a new skin care product on a small area before applying it to your entire face.

12. Consult a dermatologist: Get professional advice for persistent skin problems.

13 . Drink plenty of water: Stay hydrated for overall skin health.

14 .Eat foods rich in antioxidants: Fruits, vegetables, and green vegetables can benefit your skin.

15. Reduce sugar intake: Too much sugar can contribute to skin problems like acne.

16. Add good fats: Omega-3 fatty acids can help keep skin soft.

17. Use Vitamin C: Boost collagen production with foods rich in vitamin C.

18.Limit alcohol and caffeine: both can irritate your skin.

19. Get enough sleep: Aim for 7-9 hours of quality sleep per night.

20. Managing Stress: Stress can damage skin tissue, so engage in stress-reducing activities.

21.Regular Exercise: Regular exercise can improve blood circulation and skin health.

22.Practice good hygiene: Always wash your hands and keep your skin clean.

Some common skin problems that are prevent by following above tips:

1. Acne: A skin condition that occurs when hair follicles become clogged with oil and dead skin cells, leading to pimples, blackheads, and whiteheads.

2. Eczema: A condition that causes the skin to become inflamed, itchy, red, and cracked. It can occur in people of all ages and is often linked to allergies and asthma.

3. Dermatitis: A general term for skin inflammation that can be caused by irritants, allergens, or genetic factors. It includes conditions like contact dermatitis and seborrheic dermatitis.

4. Hives (Urticaria): Raised, red, itchy welts on the skin that often result from an allergic reaction to food, medication, or other triggers.

5. Sunburn: Skin damage caused by exposure to ultraviolet (UV) rays from the sun. It results in red, painful skin that may peel or blister.

Gut or Digestion

Stomach problems are common issues that many people experience. Here are some common stomach problems:

1. Indigestion: Also known as dyspepsia, indigestion is a term used to describe discomfort or pain in the upper abdomen. Symptoms can include bloating, belching, nausea, and a burning sensation in the upper abdomen. Indigestion can be caused by various factors, such as overeating, eating too quickly, consuming greasy or spicy foods, or stress.

2. Acid reflux: Acid reflux occurs when stomach acid flows back up into the esophagus, causing a burning sensation in the chest (heartburn) and an acidic taste in the mouth. It can be triggered by certain foods, smoking, obesity, pregnancy, or a hiatal hernia. Chronic acid reflux can lead to gastroesophageal reflux disease (GERD), a more serious condition that may require medical treatment.

3. Gastritis: Gastritis is inflammation of the stomach lining, which can be caused by various factors such as infection with Helicobacter pylori bacteria, excessive alcohol consumption, long-term use of nonsteroidal anti-inflammatory drugs (NSAIDs), stress, or autoimmune diseases. Symptoms of gastritis include abdominal pain, nausea, vomiting, bloating, and loss of appetite.

4. Peptic ulcers: Peptic ulcers are sores that develop on the lining of the stomach, small intestine, or esophagus. They can be caused by infection with H. pylori bacteria, long-term use of NSAIDs, smoking, or excessive alcohol consumption. Symptoms of peptic ulcers include burning pain in the abdomen, bloating, nausea, vomiting, and weight loss.

The stomach is essential for proper digestion and absorption of nutrients as well as maintaining the overall health and well-being of the body. Malfunctioning or diseased stomach can lead to serious digestive issues and health problems.

Good digestion is crucial for health, especially for older people. It helps the body absorb nutrients, boosts the immune system, provides energy, manages weight, supports mental health, prevents diseases, and improves comfort and quality of life.

It's important to address any digestive issues and get professional advice for personalized care.

Below are some tips for a healthy stomach and better digestion:

1. Eat a balanced diet high in fiber and rich in fruits, vegetables, and whole grains.

2. Stay hydrated by drinking plenty of water throughout the day.

3. Eat mindfully and chew your food thoroughly to aid digestion

4. Don't eat too quickly or lose focus to avoid overeating

5. Include probiotic-rich foods like yogurt, kefir, and sauerkraut in your diet.

6. Limit your intake of processed foods, refined sugars, and artificial sweeteners.

7. Include prebiotic foods like bananas, onions, and garlic in your diet to support gut health.

8.Manage stress through relaxation techniques such as meditation, yoga, and deep breathing.

9. Exercise regularly to promote healthy digestion and bowel movements.

10. Avoid excessive alcohol consumption as it can irritate the stomach lining.

11. Limit your intake of caffeine and spicy foods as they can cause heartburn.

12. Practice portion control to prevent bloating and indigestion.

13. Include healthy sources of fats like avocados, nuts, olive oil etc in your diet.

14. Eat smaller, more frequent meals throughout the day instead of larger ones.

15. Avoid eating late at night to ensure adequate digestion before bedtime.

16. Limit your intake of fatty and fried foods as they can slow down digestion.

17. Include ginger in your diet or drink ginger tea to aid digestion.

18. To aid digestion, stay active and maintain a healthy weight.

19. Avoid smoking as it can damage the digestive system and increase the risk of ulcers.

20. Limit your intake of carbonated drinks as they can cause gas and bloating.

21. Consume fermented foods such as kimchi, miso, and tempeh to promote gut health.

22. Be aware of food sensitivities and intolerances and adjust your diet accordingly.

23. To prevent heartburn and indigestion, avoid eating too close to bedtime.

24. Practice good hygiene to avoid food poisoning and stomach infections.

25. Limit your intake of artificial additives, preservatives, and processed foods.

26. Eat insoluble fiber such as whole grains and vegetables to ensure regular bowel movements.

27. Limit your intake of sugary foods and drinks as they can upset the balance of your intestinal flora.

28. Eat green leafy vegetables like spinach, kale for healthy digestion.

29. Avoid overuse of over-the-counter antacids as they can affect stomach acid levels.

30. Consume sources of soluble fiber like oats, legumes, and flaxseeds to regulate digestion.

31. Don't eat too quickly or skip meals, as this can affect your digestion.

32. Stay hydrated throughout the day with herbal teas, flavored water, or plain water.

33. If you are lactose intolerant, limit your intake of high-fat dairy products.

34. Include lean sources of protein in your diet, such as chicken, fish, and tofu.

35. Try mindful eating habits, such as keeping a food diary and saying gratitude before meals.

36. If you have a sensitive stomach, avoid eating large amounts of spicy foods.

37. Drink fermented drinks such as kombucha or kefir to reap the benefits of probiotics.

38. Practice stress-reducing activities such as yoga, meditation, and spending time in nature.

39. Avoid overuse of antibiotics as they can upset the balance of your gut flora.

40. To maintain a healthy gut flora, consume sources of resistant starch such as green bananas, cooked and cooled potatoes, and legumes.

41. If you have trouble digesting certain foods, consider taking a digestive enzyme supplement.

42. Limit your intake of artificial sweeteners such as sorbitol, as these can cause digestive problems.

43 Avoid eating close to an intense workout to prevent stomach upset.

44. Try intermittent fasting or time-restricted eating for healthy digestion.

45. Eat a variety of colorful fruits and vegetables to benefit from a range of nutrients and antioxidants.

46. Limit your intake of processed meats and foods rich in sodium, as these can cause digestive problems.

47. Ask your doctor or nutritionist for personal advice on how to improve your stomach health and digestion.

By incorporating these tips into your daily life and making conscious dietary and lifestyle choices, you can support your stomach health and promote optimal digestion. Please note that individual needs may vary, so to maintain healthy digestion and overall wellness, it is important to listen to your body and adjust your habits accordingly.

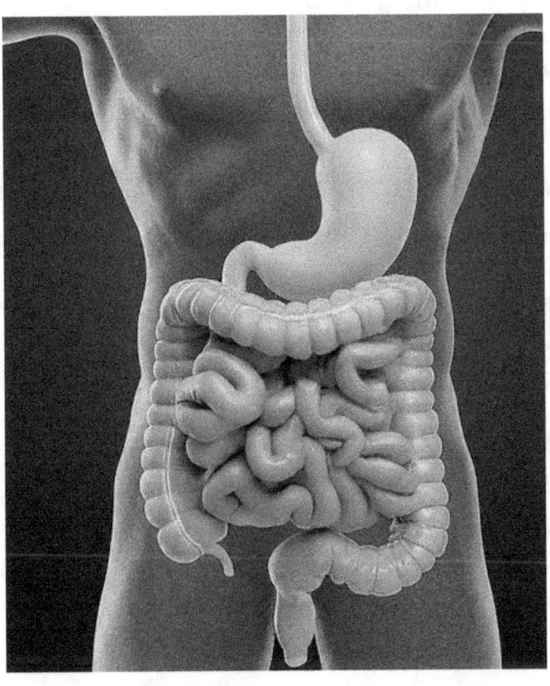

Bones and Joint

Bones and joints are a vital part of the musculoskeletal system, contributing to movement, support, protection and overall health. Maintaining bone and joint health through proper nutrition, exercise and lifestyle choices is critical to overall well-being and quality of life.

Healthy joints are crucial for mobility, flexibility and overall quality of life.

Joint problems can arise from various conditions and injuries, leading to pain, stiffness, and reduced mobility.

Osteoarthritis is the most common form of arthritis, characterized by the degeneration of cartilage in the joints. It often leads to pain, swelling, and decreased range of motion, typically affecting weight-bearing joints such as knees, hips, and the spine.

Below are some tips to help promote joint health and prevent problems like arthritis and joint pain.

1. Stay active: Regular exercise strengthens the muscles around your joints and promotes joint health.

2. Maintain a healthy weight: Being overweight puts more strain on your joints, so aim for a healthy weight.

3. Stretch Daily: Include stretching exercises to increase flexibility and reduce joint stiffness.

4. Maintain Good Posture: Good posture helps prevent joint strain and supports spinal health.

5. Eat a balanced diet: Consume foods rich in antioxidants, omega-3 fatty acids, and vitamins to support joint health.

6. Stay hydrated: Drink plenty of water to keep your joints flexible and your cartilage healthy.

7. Avoid inflammatory foods: Limit your intake of processed foods, sugary snacks, and trans fats that can cause inflammation.

8. Maintain good posture: Lift heavy objects properly and avoid repetitive movements that put strain on your joints.

9. Wear supportive shoes: Choose shoes with good arch support and cushioning to protect your joints.

10. Protect your joints: Use knee pads, wrist braces, or other protective equipment when performing high-impact activities.

11. Warm up before exercise: Always warm up with light exercise to prepare your joints for more intense exercise.

12. Cool down after exercise: Finish your exercise with light stretches to prevent muscle tension and stiff joints.

13. Listen to your body: Pay attention to any pain or discomfort in your joints and adjust your activities accordingly.

14. Practice mindful movement: Participate in activities like yoga or tai chi that promote gentle, deliberate movement for joint health.

15. Maintain proper ergonomics: Adjust your workstation to ensure proper posture and reduce stress on your joints.

16. Incorporate strength training: Build muscle strength to support joint stability and reduce the risk of injury.

17. Get adequate rest: Give your body time to recover and regenerate to support joint health.

18. Manage Stress: Practice stress reduction techniques such as meditation and deep breathing, as chronic stress can cause inflammation.

19. Avoid Smoking: Smoking can weaken bones and cartilage, leading to joint problems.

20. Consider joint-friendly supplements: Ask your doctor about supplements such as glucosamine and chondroitin for joint support.

21. Use proper lifting techniques: Lift with your legs bent at the knees to protect your back and joints.

22. Ice for painful joints: Apply ice to inflamed joints to reduce swelling and pain.

23. Use heat therapy: Apply heat to stiff joints to improve circulation and reduce stiffness.

24. Take breaks: If you have a sedentary job, take breaks to stand up, stretch, and move around to prevent stiff joints.

25. Practice good hygiene: Keep joints clean and dry to prevent infection and skin irritation.

26. Stay active throughout the day: Include short walks and stretching exercises in your daily routine to keep your joints flexible.

27. Consider low-impact exercise: Swimming, cycling and walking are gentle on your joints and help you stay mobile.

28. Practice good sleep hygiene: Get plenty of restful sleep to support joint healing and overall health.

29. Protect your joints while exercising: Wear appropriate protective clothing and warm up properly before exercising.

30. Stay informed: Learn about joint health, common symptoms like arthritis, and prevention strategies.

31. Avoid sitting for long periods of time. Get up and move around regularly to prevent stiff joints and muscle tension.

32. Use assistive devices: If needed, use ergonomic tools and equipment to reduce stress on your joints during daily activities.

33. Participate in joint-friendly activities: Choose joint-friendly activities such as swimming, yoga, pilates, etc.

34. Stay flexible: Incorporate activities such as yoga and stretching to maintain joint flexibility and range of motion.

35. Consult a Physiotherapist: Consult a physiotherapist for advice on customized exercises that promote joint health.

36.Protect your joints in cold weather: Wear warm clothing and cover your joints to prevent stiffness in cold temperatures.

37. Avoid high-impact activities: Limit activities that put undue strain on your joints, especially if you already have joint problems.

38. Maintain balance: Strengthen your core muscles to improve balance and stability, reducing the risk of falls and joint injuries.

39. Be consistent: Practice joint-friendly exercise and healthy habits regularly to maintain long-term joint health.

Brain

A healthy brain is essential for cognitive function, memory, and general well-being.

Below are some tips to support brain health and cognitive function:

1. Stay physically active: Regular exercise increases blood flow to the brain and supports cognitive function.

2. Eat a balanced diet: Eat brain-boosting foods like oily fish, nuts, seeds, fruits, and vegetables.

3. Stay Hydrated: Drink plenty of water to support brain function and prevent dehydration.

4. Get Enough Sleep: Aim for 7-9 hours of quality sleep each night to support memory consolidation and cognitive function.

5. Challenge your brain: Engage in mentally stimulating activities like puzzles, reading, learning a new skill, playing an instrument, etc.

6. Manage stress: Practice stress reduction techniques like meditation, deep breathing, and yoga to protect your brain health

7. Stay socially connected: Maintain relationships with friends and family to support your mental health and cognitive function.

8. Protect your head: Wear a helmet when playing sports to avoid head injuries and protect your head from trauma.

9. Limit your alcohol intake: Excessive alcohol consumption can affect brain function and cognitive performance.

10. Quit smoking: Smoking can damage blood vessels and reduce blood flow to the brain, affecting cognitive health.

11. Stay mentally active: To maintain cognitive function, constantly learn new things, take up hobbies and challenge your brain.

12. Maintain a healthy weight: Obesity has been linked to decreased cognitive function, so aim for a healthy weight through diet and exercise.

13. Limit Sugar and Processed Foods: A diet high in sugar and processed foods can negatively impact brain health and cognitive function.

14. Get Omega-3 Fatty Acids: Foods rich in omega-3 fatty acids, such as oily fish, flaxseeds, and walnuts, support brain health.

25. Stay Active: Regular physical activity promotes the growth of new brain cells and improves cognitive function.

16. Practice Mindfulness: Mindfulness meditation reduces stress, improves focus, and supports brain health.

17. Maintain Healthy Blood Pressure: High blood pressure can damage blood vessels in the brain and affect cognitive function.

18. Protect your hearing: Hearing loss is associated with decreased cognitive function, so protect your hearing and get treatment if necessary.

19. Get your eyes checked regularly: Poor vision can affect cognitive function, so get your eyes checked regularly.

20.Limit Exposure to Toxins: Reduce exposure to environmental toxins, pollutants, and chemicals that can harm brain health.

21. Get Organized: Use calendars, planners, and reminders to reduce cognitive load and brain stress.

22. Practice Gratitude: Practice gratitude to cultivate a positive mindset and support emotional well-being and brain health.

23. Seek support for mental health issues: Treat mental health issues such as anxiety, depression, and mood disorders to protect your brain health.

24. Stay curious: Be curious, ask questions, and seek out new experiences to keep your brain busy and active.

25. Limit screen time: Excessive screen time can affect cognitive function. Therefore, take regular breaks and limit your use.

26. Stay educated: Continue learning throughout your life to challenge your brain and support cognitive function.

27. Protect your brain: Wear a seat belt in the car, wear a helmet when exercising, and take precautions to prevent head injuries.

28. Maintain good posture: Good posture promotes spinal health, which in turn leads to brain health and cognitive function.

29. Participate in creative activities: Stimulate your brain and explore your creativity through art, music, writing and other creative activities.

30. Maintain good oral health: Oral health is linked to brain health, so make dental hygiene a priority.

31. Limit caffeine and alcohol: Excessive caffeine and alcohol intake can affect sleep quality and cognitive function.

32. Get regular medical checkups: Regular medical checkups can identify problems that may affect brain health, such as: High cholesterol or high blood pressure.

33. Stay Positive: Maintain a positive attitude, value yourself, and surround yourself with supportive relationships.

34. Practice Deep Breathing: Practicing deep breathing can reduce stress, improve focus, and promote brain health.

35. Stay Informed: Stay up to date on brain health research, cognitive training, and strategies to maintain cognitive function.

36. Limit Noise Exposure: Protect your hearing from loud noises that can affect your cognitive health.

37. Get Mentally Active: Keep your brain sharp by participating in brain teasers, puzzles, memory games, and other cognitive challenges.

38. Maintain a healthy gut: Gut health is linked to brain health, so include probiotic-rich foods and fiber in your diet.

39. Get organized: Use a calendar, planner, or to-do list to reduce cognitive load and stay on track.

40. Exercise your brain power: Take part in activities that challenge your memory, attention, and cognitive skills to promote brain health.

41. Limit your exposure to air pollution: Air pollution can affect your brain health. Therefore, avoid areas with high levels of air pollution as much as possible.

42. Practice mindful eating: Be mindful of your food choices, enjoy flavors and eat mindfully to support your overall health, including your brain health.

43. Maintain healthy relationships: Positive social connections promote brain health and mental well-being.

44. Limit processed foods: Processed foods high in additives, preservatives and artificial ingredients can have a negative impact on brain health.

45. Practice time management: Prioritize tasks, set goals and manage your time effectively to reduce stress and support brain function.

46. Seek mental stimulation: Read a book, solve a puzzle, play a brain game, or take part in a cognitively stimulating activity.

47. Eat foods rich in antioxidants: Foods high in antioxidants, such as berries, dark chocolate, and leafy greens, protect brain cells from damage.

48. Treat chronic conditions: Manage chronic conditions such as diabetes, high blood pressure, and high cholesterol that can affect brain health.

49. Maintain hygiene: Wash your hands regularly, practice good hygiene, and avoid contact with germs that can cause infections and affect brain health.

50. Visit your healthcare provider: Visit your healthcare provider regularly for tests, exams, and consultations to monitor and support your brain health.

By incorporating these tips into your daily life and making proactive decisions to support your brain health, you can improve your cognitive function, memory, and overall brain health. Remember, lifestyle factors, diet, mental stimulation, and social contact all play an important role in maintaining a healthy brain throughout your life. It's not too late to start implementing these strategies and prioritize your brain health for a fulfilling, vibrant life.

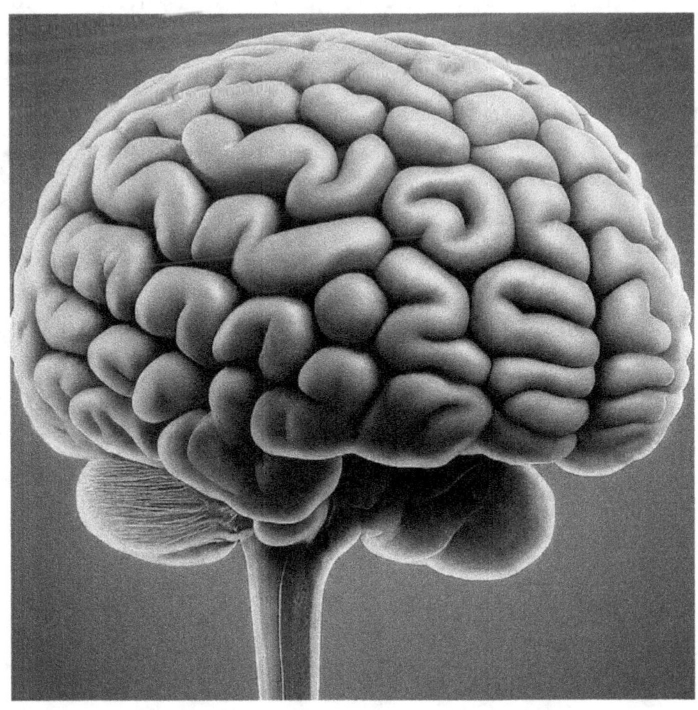

Heart

The heart is extremely important because it pumps oxygen-rich blood throughout the body. This vital organ supports cellular function, regulates blood pressure, and removes waste products. Maintaining a healthy heart through diet, exercise, and regular checkups is critical to your overall health.

Some tips for a healthy heart:

1. Maintain a healthy weight.

2. Be physically active and exercise regularly.

3. Eat a balanced diet and include plenty of fruits, vegetables, whole grains, and lean proteins.

4. Avoid processed foods that are high in sugar, salt, and unhealthy fats.

5. Limit your intake of red meat and choose lean proteins.

6. Include heart-healthy fats in your diet, such as omega-3 fatty acids.

7. Reduce your intake of saturated and trans fats.

8. Limit your intake of sugary drinks and high-calorie snacks.

9. Monitor your cholesterol levels and keep them under control.

10. Control your blood pressure through diet, exercise, and medication, if necessary.

11. Manage your stress levels through relaxation and mindfulness exercises.

12. Get regularly checked for risk factors for heart disease.

13. Avoid smoking and exposure to passive smoking.

14. Limit alcohol intake to moderate levels.

15. Stay hydrated by drinking plenty of water.

16. Get enough sleep to maintain a healthy heart.

17. Maintain good oral hygiene to reduce the risk of heart disease.

18. Participate in hobbies and activities that bring you joy and reduce stress.

19. Avoid sitting for long periods of time and take breaks to move around physically throughout the day.

20. Control your portion sizes to manage your calorie intake.

21. Track your food intake and physical activity to maintain a healthy lifestyle.

22. Participate in activities that promote social connections and mental well-being.

23. If you have diabetes or are at risk for diabetes, monitor your blood sugar levels.

24. Consider incorporating meditation or yoga into your daily life to manage stress.

25. Cook your meals at home using fresh ingredients to control food quality.

26. Plan your meals and snacks in advance to avoid unhealthy choices.

27. Use herbs and spices to season your foods instead of relying on salt.

28. Include nuts and seeds in your diet to get heart-healthy fats and fiber.

29. Choose whole grains, such as brown rice, quinoa and oats, instead of refined grains.

30. Limit your intake of processed meats, such as bacon and sausages.

31. Choose low-fat or fat-free dairy products to reduce your intake of saturated fat.

32. Include a variety of colorful fruits and vegetables in your diet to get a variety of nutrients.

33. Enjoy your food, pay attention to your hunger cues, and practice mindful eating.

34. Read food labels to identify hidden sources of sugar, salt, and unhealthy fats.

35. Cook with heart-healthy oils, such as olive oil or avocado oil.

36. Limit fast food and restaurant meals high in sodium and unhealthy fats.

37. Stay active throughout the day by taking short walks, stretching, and using a standing desk.

38. Set realistic physical activity goals and track your progress.

39. Join a fitness class or group activity to stay motivated and committed.

40. Incorporate strength training into your daily routine to improve your heart health.

41. Practice breathing exercises to reduce stress and promote relaxation.

42. Limit screen time and prioritize personal interactions with friends and family.

43. Volunteer or serve your community to support your mental health.

44. Practice gratitude by expressing gratitude for the positive aspects of life.

45. Stay up to date on heart health research and recommendations.

46. If you are experiencing emotional problems, consider seeking the support of a therapist or counselor.

47. Prioritize self-care activities such as reading, listening to music, or taking a bath.

48. Stay connected with your loved ones through phone calls, video chats, or in-person visits.

49. Engage in a creative hobby, such as painting, gardening or crafting, to reduce stress.

50. Celebrate progress and achievements on your journey to a healthy heart.

Please note that these tips are general guidelines and you should always consult with your doctor before making any major changes to your lifestyle or diet.

Lungs

The lungs are vital organs responsible for gas exchange, bringing oxygen into the bloodstream and excreting carbon dioxide. They play a key role in maintaining the body's pH balance and support cellular respiration. Healthy lungs are vital to overall health and enable physical activity and endurance. Proper care, including avoiding smoking and pollution, is crucial for lung function and longevity.

Some tips for Healthy Lungs:

1. Quit smoking :
The most important step for your lung health is to quit smoking. Smoking damages lung tissue and increases your risk of lung disease.

2. Avoid passive smoking :
Stay away from places where smoking is occurring. Secondhand smoke can be just as harmful as smoking itself.

3. Stay active :
   Exercise regularly. Exercise strengthens your respiratory muscles and improves lung capacity.

4. Practice deep breathing :
Incorporate deep breathing into your daily routine. This helps expand your lungs and improves oxygen absorption.

5. Maintain a healthy weight :
Obesity can affect lung function. Eat a balanced diet and exercise regularly to maintain a healthy weight.

6. Stay hydrated :
Drink plenty of water to keep the lining of your lungs moist, helping
it trap dust and bacteria.

7. Eat a balanced diet Include fruits, vegetables, whole grains, and
lean proteins in your diet. The antioxidants in these foods may help
protect lung tissue.

8. Limit your exposure to air pollution
Try to avoid areas with high levels of air pollution. If you live in a
polluted area, consider using an air purifier indoors.

9. Get regular medical checkups :
 Make sure to see your doctor for regular checkups to monitor your
lung health, especially if you have a history of respiratory illness.

10. Maintain good hygiene :To prevent respiratory infections, wash
your hands frequently. Avoid close contact with people who are
sick.

11. Get vaccinated :To protect yourself against respiratory
infections, keep your vaccinations up to date, including flu and
pneumonia shots.

12. Avoid Allergens:Identify allergens, such as dust, mold, and pet
dander, that can cause respiratory problems and minimize your
exposure to them.

13. Use a Humidifier :Keep the humidity in your home at an optimum
to avoid dry air that can irritate your lungs.

14. Limit caffeine and alcohol :Consuming too much caffeine or
alcohol can cause dehydration and affect lung function.

15. Do yoga :yoga improves lung capacity and promotes relaxation
through controlled breathing techniques.

16. Avoid overexertion :
Listen to your body and try not to push yourself too hard during physical activity, especially if you already have lung problems.

17. Wear protective clothing :
If you work in an environment with dust, chemicals, or pollutants, wear a mask or respirator to protect your lungs.

18. Limit processed foods :
Reduce your intake of processed foods high in sugar and unhealthy fats, as they can cause inflammation.

19. Eat Omega-3 Fatty Acids :
Foods rich in omega-3 fatty acids, such as fish, flaxseeds, and walnuts, can help reduce lung inflammation.

20. Avoid Cold Air :
Cold air can narrow your airways. If you exercise outdoors in the winter, cover your mouth with a scarf.

21. Watch Your Posture :
Good posture improves lung capacity. Sit or stand upright so your lungs can fully expand.

22. Limit Your Milk Intake :
Some people feel that dairy products can increase mucus production. If this happens to you, watch your intake.

23. Use essential oils :
Certain essential oils, such as eucalyptus and peppermint, can help open airways and improve breathing.

24. Get aerobic exercise :
Activities such as running, swimming, and cycling can improve lung capacity and performance.

25. Avoid Excessive Coughing
Chronic coughing can irritate the lungs. If you are suffering from a
persistent cough, see a doctor.

26. Manage Stress :
High levels of stress can affect your breathing patterns. Practice
relaxation techniques such as meditation and mindfulness.

27. Limit Exposure to Chemicals :
Minimize contact with household cleaners and chemicals. Choose
natural alternatives where possible.

28. Get Enough Sleep :
Adequate sleep is essential for overall health, including lung
function. Aim for 7-9 hours of restful sleep each night.

29. Stay Updated :
 Learn about lung health and stay up to date on new research and
recommendations.

30. Avoid Excessive Heat :
Hot, humid air can make it hard to breathe. In hot weather, stay cool
and drink plenty of fluids.

31. Use nasal sprays :
If you suffer from allergies, you should use saline nasal sprays to
keep your nasal passages clear.

32. Limit time indoors :
Avoid spending long periods of time in crowded, enclosed spaces
where airborne diseases can spread.

33. Use spices :
Spices such as turmeric and ginger have anti-inflammatory
properties that may have a positive impact on lung health.

34. Monitor air quality :
Check local air quality reports and limit outdoor activities if air pollution levels are high.

35. Avoid excessive talking :
If you have a sore throat or difficulty breathing, you should limit your talking to avoid straining your vocal cords and lungs.

36. Use a face mask :
Wearing a mask can help protect your lungs if you live in an area with high air pollution or during flu season.

37. Limit your sugar intake :
Excessive sugar intake can cause inflammation. Choose natural sweeteners whenever possible.

38. Do breathing exercises :
Introduce exercises such as lip braking to improve lung function and oxygen delivery.

39. Stay in touch :
Maintaining social contact to promote mental health may indirectly have a positive impact on lung health.

40. Avoid Excessive Alcohol Intake :
Limit your alcohol intake as excessive alcohol consumption can weaken your immune system and affect your lung health.

41. Use Natural Cleaners :
Choose environmentally friendly cleaning products to reduce your exposure to harmful chemicals.

42. Eat fiber :
A diet high in fiber reduces inflammation and improves lung function.

43. Stay positive : A positive attitude improves overall health, including lung health. Practice gratitude and mindfulness.

44. Limit Screen Time :
Excessive screen time can lead to a sedentary lifestyle. Take breaks and exercise.

45. Avoid Over-the-Counter Medications
Limit your use of over-the-counter medications that can dry out your airways.
46. Stay up to date on lung diseases
 Learn about lung diseases and their symptoms to identify problems early.

47. Seek professional help
If respiratory symptoms persist, contact your doctor for a diagnosis.

48. Limit exposure to cold air
If you have asthma or other respiratory diseases, avoid exposure to cold air as it can trigger symptoms.

49. Get Involved in Community Activities
Participate in local activities that promote health and wellness, such as lung health education.

50. Pay Attention to Your Breath
Practice mindfulness and pay attention to your breathing patterns. This can help manage stress and improve lung function.

Kidney

Kidneys are important organs for maintaining overall health. They filter waste and excess fluid from the blood, regulate electrolyte balance, and help control blood pressure. In addition, kidneys produce hormones that are very important for red blood cell production and bone health. Normal kidney function is essential for the body to excrete and maintain hydration and electrolyte levels.

Some tips for healthy Kidneys:

1. Stay hydrated: Drinking plenty of water helps the kidneys remove waste.

2 .Reduce sodium: Reduce salt intake to help control blood pressure.

3 .Eat fresh fruits and vegetables: They are rich in vitamins and minerals.

4 .Choose whole grains: Choose whole grains instead of refined grains.

5. Limit processed foods: These foods often contain high amounts of sodium and unhealthy fats.

6. Watch your protein intake: Too much protein can put a strain on your kidneys.

7.Reduce phosphorus: A diet high in phosphorus can be harmful

8. Healthy fats: Use healthy fats like olive oil and avocado instead of saturated fats.

9. Avoid sugary drinks: Limit soda and other sugary drinks to reduce your risk of kidney damage.

10. Maintain a healthy weight: Being overweight increases your risk of kidney disease.

11. Exercise regularly: Get at least 150 minutes of moderate exercise a week.

12. Quit smoking: Smoking can worsen kidney function and overall health.

13 Cut back on alcohol: Drink in moderation, as drinking too much can damage your kidneys.

14. Manage stress: Practice relaxation techniques such as yoga or meditation.

15.Regular visits to your health care provider can help monitor kidney health.

16.Keep your blood pressure in a healthy range.

17.Control your blood sugar levels: If you have diabetes, manage your blood sugar levels properly.

18.Know your family history: Be aware of any family history of kidney disease.

19. Get kidney function tests: Regular checkups can help detect problems early.

20.Use medications wisely: Follow your doctor's advice when taking medications, especially NSAIDs.

21.Avoid over-the-counter pain relievers: Limit the use of ibuprofen and naproxen because they can harm your kidneys.

22.Check before taking supplements: Some supplements can affect kidney function, always check with your healthcare provider.

23. Drink water before eating: This helps with hydration and digestion.

24. Limit caffeine: Consuming too much caffeine can lead to dehydration.

25. Use herbs and spices: Use herbs and spices instead of salt in foods.

26.Cooking at home: Preparing meals at home allows you to control ingredients and portion sizes.

27.Read food labels: Check the sodium and phosphorus content of packaged foods.

28. Get informed: Learn about kidney health and disease prevention.

29. Join a support group: Connect with others for support and information.

30. Reduce exposure to toxins and chemicals.

31. Pregnancy and kidney health: Pregnant women should carefully monitor the health of their kidneys.

32. Age Considerations: Kidney function naturally declines with age.

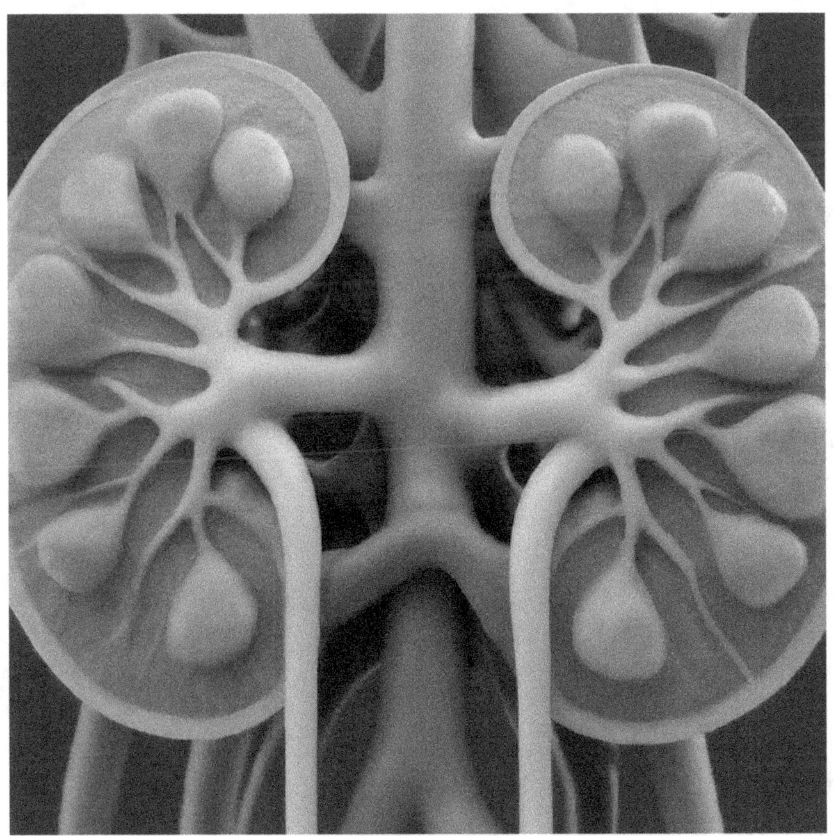

Good Sleep

A good night's sleep is important for your health as a whole. It improves mood, immune system strength, and cognitive function. Sleeping well promotes emotional regulation and memory consolidation. Sleep is an essential part of daily wellness because it can improve productivity and quality of life, making it a priority.

Some few tips for good Sleep are as follows:

1. Keep a regular sleeping schedule by going to bed and getting up at the same time each day, even on weekends.

2. Establish a Calming Bedtime Routine: Before going to bed, engage in calming activities like reading, meditating, or taking a warm bath.

3. Limit Screen Time: Avoid using screens (phones, tablets, or computers) for at least an hour before going to bed because blue light can make your body produce less melatonin.

4. Improve Your Sleep Environment: Make sure your bedroom is cool, dark, and quiet. Consider power outage drapes, earplugs, or a background noise.

5. Make an investment in a mattress and pillows that are both supportive and comfortable for your sleeping position.

6. Limit Caffeine and Nicotine: Avoid caffeine and nicotine just before bedtime because they can make it hard to sleep.

7. Maintain a healthy diet by avoiding large meals, spicy foods, and excessive liquids just before bedtime to avoid discomfort and frequent bathroom breaks.

8. Exercise on a regular basis: Try to avoid doing strenuous exercise right before bedtime.

9. Oversee Pressure and Tension: Practice unwinding methods like profound breathing, yoga, or care to lessen pressure before bed.

10. Limit Naps: If you have to take a nap, keep it short (between 20 and 30 minutes) and don't take it too late in the day.

11. Increase your exposure to natural light by spending time outside during the day to help your circadian rhythm.

12. Use Your Bed Only for Sleeping: To strengthen the mental connection between your bed and sleep, don't work, eat, or watch TV in bed.

13. Melatonin and other sleep aids should be discussed with a healthcare professional if necessary.

14. Keep a sleep diary to keep track of your sleep habits, patterns, and feelings to find things that might be affecting your sleep.

15. Limit your intake of alcohol: Although alcohol may assist you in falling asleep, it can disrupt your circadian rhythms during the night.

16. Remain Hydrated: Hydrate over the course of the day, yet limit admission near sleep time to keep away from evening enlightenments.

17. Look for Proficient Assistance if necessary: On the off chance that you reliably battle with rest, consider counseling a rest expert for assessment and direction.

18. To cultivate a more upbeat outlook, practice gratitude by taking a few minutes before going to bed to think about experiences or things for which you are grateful.

19. Use Fragrant healing: Consider utilizing quieting fragrances like lavender or chamomile to make a relieving climate.

20. Be Aware of Rest Problems: Know about indications of rest issues, like a sleeping disorder or rest apnea, and look for proficient assistance in the event that you suspect you might have one.

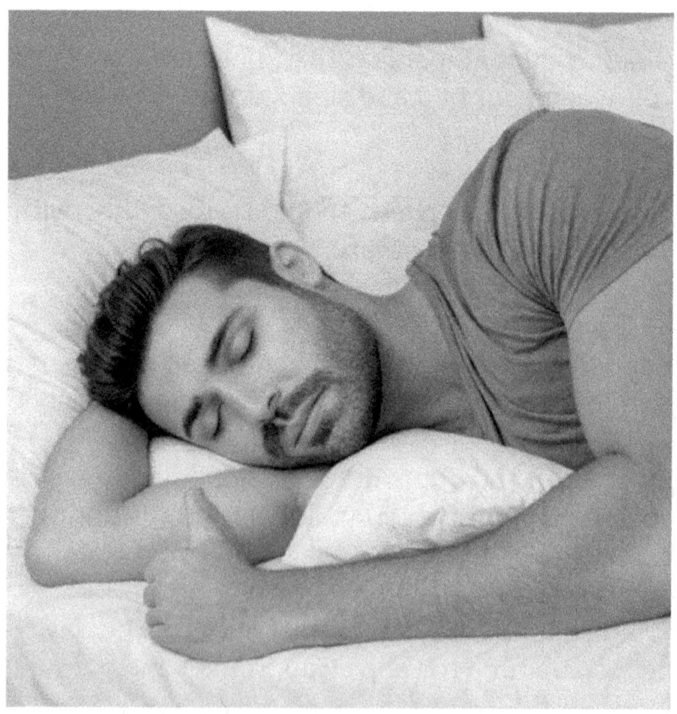

Dental care

Maintaining excellent dental care is vital for keeping the body healthy and avoiding problems with teeth. Consistent brushing and flossing aid in getting rid of plaque, which lowers the chance of getting cavities and gum disease. Moreover, taking good care of your mouth can stop bad breath and make your teeth look whiter. More than just looking good, having good dental care is connected to the overall well-being of the body, since poor dental health can lead to diseases such as heart disease and diabetes. Going for regular dental appointments also helps in spotting issues early on, making dental care a key component of a healthy way of living.

Below are some good tips to maintain proper oral hygiene.

1. Brush Your Teeth Twice a Day: Make it a habit to brush your teeth at least twice daily, ideally in the morning and before going to sleep.

2. Choose Fluoride Toothpaste: Select a toothpaste that contains fluoride to strengthen your tooth enamel and prevent cavities.

3. Floss Every Day: Floss at the very least once daily to remove plaque and food debris from the spaces between your teeth that a toothbrush can't reach.

4. Rinse with an Antimicrobial Mouthwash: Use an antimicrobial mouthwash to help decrease plaque, gingivitis, and combat bad breath.

5. Replace Your Toothbrush Every 3-4 Months: Change your toothbrush every 3-4 months or earlier if the bristles start to wear out.

6. Brush for Two Minutes: Spend at least two minutes brushing your teeth to ensure you clean all areas thoroughly.

7. Employ Correct Brushing Techniques: Hold your toothbrush at a 45-degree angle to your gums and use soft, circular strokes.

8. Clean Your Tongue: Gently brush your tongue or use a tongue scraper to remove bacteria and freshen your breath.

9. Cut Back on Sugary Foods and Drinks: Reduce your consumption of sugary snacks and drinks, which can lead to tooth decay.

10. Drink Plenty of Water: Stay hydrated by drinking lots of water throughout the day to help wash away food particles and bacteria.

11. Incorporate Healthy Foods: Include a variety of fruits, vegetables, whole grains, and dairy products in your diet to promote oral health.

12. Avoid Tobacco Use: Smoking and chewing tobacco can cause gum disease, tooth decay, and oral cancer.

13. Chew Sugar-Free Gum: Chewing sugar-free gum can stimulate saliva flow, which helps protect against cavities.

14. See Your Dentist Regularly: Schedule appointments for dental check-ups and cleanings at least twice a year for professional care.

15. Consider Dental Sealants: Discuss with your dentist about getting dental sealants for an additional layer of cavity protection.

16. Use Whitening Products Wisely: Follow the instructions for whitening products and consult your dentist to prevent enamel damage.

17. Wear a Mouthguard: If you participate in sports or grind your teeth at night, wearing a mouthguard can safeguard your teeth.

18. Limit Alcohol Intake: Too much alcohol can cause dry mouth and increase the risk of oral health problems.

19. Address Dry Mouth: Talk to your dentist about solutions for dry mouth, such as using saliva substitutes.

20. Learn More About Oral Health: Stay informed about oral health and hygiene practices to make informed decisions about your dental care.

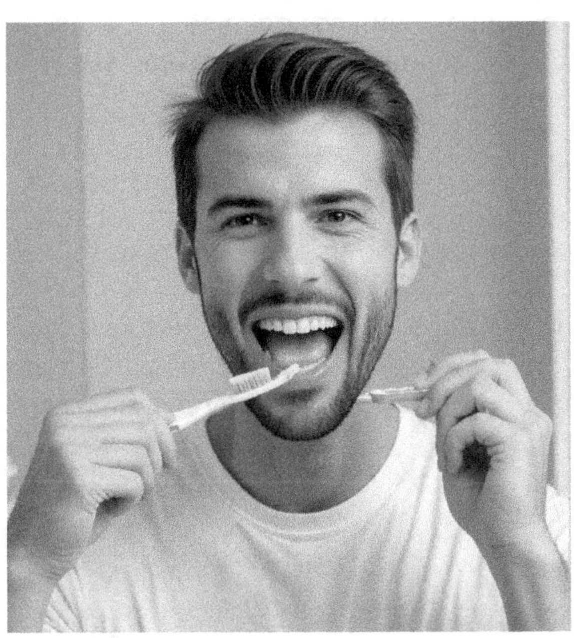

Strong Immunity

Immunity is the body's protective barrier against infections and diseases. Having a strong defense system is key to keeping healthy and feeling good. It guards against harmful microorganisms such as bacteria, viruses, and molds, stopping sickness and infections.

A powerful defense system is also crucial for identifying and getting rid of rogue cells, lowering the chance of long-term health issues, like cancer. Moreover, resistance aids in the healing process, helping the body recover more efficiently from sickness or injury.

Things like diet, exercise, rest, and managing stress greatly affect the immune system's performance. A well-rounded diet full of essential vitamins and minerals, consistent physical activity, enough sleep, and proper stress handling can boost resistance.

Some tips for healthy immune system are as follows:

1. Maintain a Nutrient-Rich Diet: Include a variety of fresh produce, whole grains, lean meats, and heart-healthy fats to ensure you're getting all the necessary vitamins and minerals.

2. Keep Hydrated: Drink enough water throughout the day to support your body's natural functions.

3. Engage in Regular Physical Activity: Aim for at least 150 minutes of moderate-intensity exercise or 75 minutes of vigorous activity weekly.

4. Prioritize Rest: Get between 7 to 9 hours of deep sleep each night to help your immune system stay strong.

5. Reduce Stress Levels: Use relaxation methods like meditation, yoga, or deep breathing to lower stress.

6. Keep Your Weight in Check: Work towards and keep your weight within a healthy range to bolster your immune system.

7. Cut Back on Added Sugars and Processed Meals: Minimize your sugar intake and avoid highly processed foods to protect your immune health.

8. Add Probiotics to Your Diet: Eat fermented foods such as yogurt, kefir, sauerkraut, and kimchi to improve gut health.

9. Ensure Adequate Vitamin D Intake: Spend time outdoors or consider taking supplements since vitamin D is vital for immune function.

10. Consume Foods Rich in Antioxidants: Eat berries, nuts, and dark chocolate to fight off oxidative damage.

11. Include Garlic and Ginger in Your Meals: These ingredients offer natural anti-inflammatory and immune-enhancing benefits.

12. Keep Up with Vaccinations: Make sure to get the recommended vaccines to protect against various illnesses.

13. Moderate Alcohol Use: Too much alcohol can weaken your immune system, so drink responsibly.

14. Quit Smoking: Smoking can harm your immune system and make you more prone to infections.

15. Practice Good Hygiene Habits: Wash your hands frequently and maintain cleanliness to avoid getting sick.

16. Enjoy Time in Nature: Being outdoors can boost your mood and overall health.

17. Stay Connected with People: Keep in touch with friends and family as positive relationships can improve your emotional health and immunity.

18. Explore Herbal Remedies: Certain herbs like echinacea and elderberry might support your immune system, but it's important to talk to a healthcare professional before trying them.

19. Limit Your Caffeine Intake: Too much caffeine can interfere with sleep and increase stress, so drink it in moderation.

20. Listen to Your Body's Needs: Pay attention to feelings of fatigue or illness and take the time to rest and recover when necessary.

Look Young

The Value of Being Young

Being young is frequently linked with vigor, enthusiasm, and a new way of seeing the world. It's essential for personal growth and a healthy life. Adopting a youthful attitude boosts creativity and flexibility, helping people face obstacles with a hopeful attitude.

Furthermore, a young perspective promotes continuous learning and discovery, which improves mental sharpness and toughness. It also strengthens social ties, as young people usually participate more in their communities.

At its core, cultivating a youthful spirit can result in a more rewarding and lively existence, no matter one's age. It encourages us to value curiosity, welcome change, and keep a positive attitude, which in turn enhances our experiences and connections with others.

1. Keep an Open Mind: Foster a sense of curiosity and wonder about the world around you. Ask questions and seek out new experiences.

2. Continue to Learn: Engage in learning throughout your life. Try new hobbies, sign up for classes, or dive into books on a variety of topics.

3. Exercise Regularly: Stay active by engaging in consistent physical activity. Discover an exercise routine that you enjoy, whether it's dancing, hiking, or practicing yoga.

4. Eat Healthily: Fuel your body with a diet abundant in fruits, vegetables, whole grains, and lean proteins. Remember to stay hydrated!

5. Prioritize Sleep: Make quality sleep a priority to allow your body to rest and rejuvenate.

6. Maintain Strong Social Connections: Keep in touch with friends and family, and also seek out new social connections.

7. Focus on the Positive: Concentrate on the good things in your life. Keeping a gratitude journal can help you shift your perspective towards positivity.

8. Manage Stress Effectively: Find healthy strategies to cope with stress, such as meditation, deep breathing exercises, or spending time in nature.

9. Be Open to Change: Embrace new experiences and changes. Being adaptable is crucial for maintaining a youthful outlook.

10. Find Joy in Laughter: Look for humor in everyday situations. Laughter is a powerful tool for reducing stress and improving your mood.

11. Engage in Playful Activities: Participate in fun activities, whether they're games, sports, or creative endeavors. Remember, life should be taken lightly!

12. Explore New Places: Travel and immerse yourself in different cultures and environments. Traveling can expand your horizons and revitalize your spirit.

13. Be Conscious of Screen Time: Be aware of how much time you spend on screens, especially on social media. Focus more on real-life interactions.

14. Give Back: Helping others can bring a sense of purpose and fulfillment, keeping your spirit youthful.

15. Maintain a Positive Attitude: Cultivate a positive outlook on life. Surround yourself with positive influences and avoid negativity.

16. Find Ways to Express Yourself: Discover creative outlets for self-expression, whether it's through art, writing, music, or other mediums.

17. Wear What Makes You Feel Good: Choose clothes that reflect your personality and make you feel confident, regardless of what's in fashion.

18. Take on New Challenges: Step out of your comfort zone and tackle new challenges. This can lead to personal growth and a more alive feeling.

19. Be Mindful of the Present: Stay present in the moment. Practicing mindfulness can deepen your appreciation for life and reduce stress.

20. Celebrate Your Accomplishments: Acknowledge and celebrate your achievements, no matter how small. This will foster a sense of accomplishment and joy.

By incorporating these strategies into your everyday life, you can nurture a youthful mindset and lead a vibrant, fulfilling existence at any age!

Superfoods

Superfood supplements offer extraordinary medical advantages, making them essential for a reasonable eating routine. Plentiful in nutrients, minerals, antioxidant, and healthy fats, these food sources can generally improve prosperity and assist with forestalling persistent illnesses. Superfoods like salmon, kale, blueberries, and quinoa can support heart health, improve digestion, and give you more energy. Additionally, their anti-inflammatory properties aid in improved immune function. People can make significant progress toward achieving optimal health and vitality by prioritizing superfoods, ensuring a more vibrant and active lifestyle. Take advantage of superfoods for a better future!

List of easily available Superfoods that nourish your system .

1. Blueberries
2. Kale
3. Salmon
4. Chia seeds
5. Quinoa
6. Spinach
7. Avocado
8. Almonds
9. Sweet potatoes
10. Greek yogurt
11. Oats
12. Broccoli
13. Green tea
14. Flaxseeds

15. Walnuts
16. Dark chocolate (at least 70% cocoa)
17. Garlic
18. Turmeric
19. Oranges
20. Strawberries
21. Black beans
22. Lentils
23. Pumpkin seeds
24. Beets
25. Cabbage
26. Ginger
27. Cinnamon
28. Kiwifruit
29. Pomegranate
30. Brazil nuts
31. Brussels sprouts
32. Barley
33. Swiss chard
34. Maca
35. Acai berries
36. Hemp seeds
37. Mackerel
38. Sardines
39. Seaweed
40. Papaya
41. Watercress
42. Cranberries
43. Asparagus
44. Artichokes
45. Moringa
46. Camu camu
47. Goji berries
48. Pistachios
49. Cauliflower
50. Elderberries

Asanas or Yoga

Asanas of yoga poses are a fundamental part of yoga practice. They not only increase the flexibility and strength of the body but also promote mental clarity and emotional stability. Here are some common types of asanas and their meanings:

1. Standing asanas
- Examples: Tadasana (Mountain Pose), Virabhadrasana (Warrior Pose), Trikonasana (Triangle Pose)
- Importance: These poses strengthen the legs, improve balance and increase focus. They also help with grounding and connecting to the earth.

 2. Seated Asanas
- Examples: Sukhasana (Easy Pose), Padmasana (Lotus Pose), Dandasana (Stick Pose)
- Importance: Seated poses promote stability and calm, making them ideal for meditation. They also improve flexibility in the hips and lower back.

3. Forward Bends
- Examples: Paschimottanasana (Seated Forward Bend), Uttanasana (Standing Forward Bend)
- Importance: These asanas stretch the spine and hamstrings, promote relaxation, and relieve stress and anxiety.

 4. Backbends
- Examples: Bhujangasana (Cobra Pose), Urdhva Mukha Svanasana (Upward Facing Dog), Ustrasana (Camel Pose)
- Importance: Backbends open the chest and heart, increase spinal flexibility and energize the body. They can also improve mood and self-confidence.

5. Twists
- Examples: Ardha Matsyendrasana (Half King of the Fishes Pose),
Bharadvajasana (Bharadvaja Twist)
- Importance: Twists support detoxification, improve digestion
and increase spinal mobility. It also promotes mental clarity and
focus.

6. Inversions
- Examples: Adho Mukha Svanasana (Downward Facing Dog),
Sirsasana (Headstand), Sarvangasana (Shoulderstand)
- Importance: Inversions improve blood circulation, increase
energy levels and give you a new perspective. They also help calm
the mind and reduce stress.

7. Restorative Asanas
- Example: Balasana (Child's Pose), Supta Baddha Konasana
(Reclining Angle Pose)
- Importance: These postures promote deep relaxation and
restoration. They help reduce stress and restore balance to the
body and mind.

8. Balancing Asanas
- Example: Vrksasana (Tree Pose), Garudasana (Eagle Pose)
- Meaning: Balanced postures increase stability, coordination and
focus. They also strengthen the core and improve overall body
awareness.

9. Core Strengthening Asanas
- Example: Navasana (Boat Pose), Plank Pose
- Importance: These asanas strengthen the abdominal muscles,
improve posture, and increase overall stability and balance.

10. Meditative Asanas
- Example: Siddhasana (Perfect Pose), Vajrasana (Thunderbolt Pose)
- Importance: These poses are meditative and promote calmness and focus. They help to calm the mind and increase mindfulness.

Conclusion: Practicing a variety of asanas allows for a balanced yoga practice that strengthens the body, mind and spirit. Each type of asana serves a unique purpose and contributes to overall well-being, making yoga a holistic approach to health. With regular practice, you can improve your physical strength, mental clarity, emotional resilience and spiritual growth.

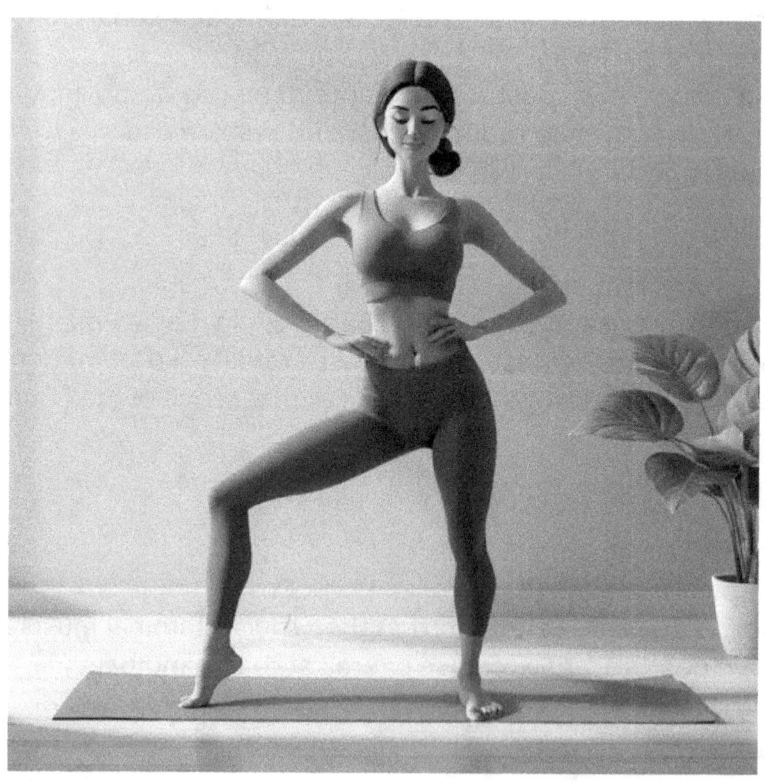

How To Stay Healthy In Rainy Season

Rainy season is imperative to maintain a strategic distance from contaminants that are common amid this time.

Below are 50 tips to assist you remain absent from diseases amid the blustery season:

1. Remain hydrated by drinking adequate amount of water.

2. Wash your hands habitually with cleanser and water.

3. Dodge streer food and eat home made cooked meals.

4. Utilize mosquito repellent to avoid mosquito-borne infections.

5. Keep your environment clean to avoid breeding grounds for mosquitoes.

6. Get immunized against common diseases like flu.

7. Maintain a strategic distance from strolling in stagnant water to avoid contaminations.
8. Utilize an umbrella or raincoat when going out within the rain.

9. Dry your feet completely in case they get damp.

10. Maintain a strategic distance from touching your face,nose with unwashed hands.

11. Boost your immune system by eating a balanaced healthy diet.
12. Get sufficient sleep and rest for better immunity .

13. Dodge crowded and congested places to diminish the hazard of presentation to contaminations.
14. Work out frequently to remain fit and boost your immune system.

15. Utilize a hand sanitizer when cleanser and water are not accessible.

16. Keep your living spaces well ventilated to anticipate any microbial growth.
17. Guarantee that your immunizations are up to date.
18. Dodge sharing individual things like towels and utensils.
19. Wear suitable footwear to ensure your feet from diseases.

20. Dry wet dress and shoes appropriately before using them.

21. Utilize clean and dry towels to maintain a strategic distance from skin diseases.

22. Utilize clean ,boiled and purified water for drinking and cooking.

23. Clean and purify habitually touched surfaces.

24. Incorporate immune-boosting foods like natural products and vegetables in your daily meals .

25. Dodge self-medication and counsel a healthcare proficient in the event that required.

26. Keep first aid kit always with you in an emergency.

27. Dodge utilizing moist or smelly towels.

28. Seek medical help if you feel sick.

29. Wash Fruits and vegetables before using them.

30. Utilize a great quality veil to anticipate the spread of respiratory contaminations.

31. Cover your mouth while coughing and sneezing to maintain good hygiene.

32. Maintain a strategic distance from sick people because disease spread more quickly in rainy season.

33. Don't eat raw or undercooked meals.

34. Keep up a secure separate from pets and animlas to anticipate contaminations.

35. Take showers after getting damp within the rain.

36. Keep your intestine healthy by consuming probiotic-rich foods.

37. Don't go out if there is a risk of heavy rain,storm and flooding.

38. Keep your windows closed amid heavy rain and storm to prevent from infection coming in your house.

39. In the rainy season, cover cooked foods to prevent infection.

40. Take a bath in Luke's warm water to unwind your body.

41. Always keep your home clean.

42. Always wear a face mask when outdoors. 43. In the rainy season, older people and children are more likely to get sick, so take good care of them.

44. It's important to protect your area during the rainy season to avoid flooding, water damage, and other problems caused by too much rain.

45 .During the rainy season, here are some tips to protect your area: Guarantee that channels and drains are clear of trash to permit water to openly stream.

46. Drains that are blocked can build up water, which can result in flooding. Removing any overhanging tree branches that could fall on your property in strong winds or rain is a good idea.

47. Keep an eye on the weather and be ready for a lot of rain. Keep up with any warnings or alerts that are going on in your area.

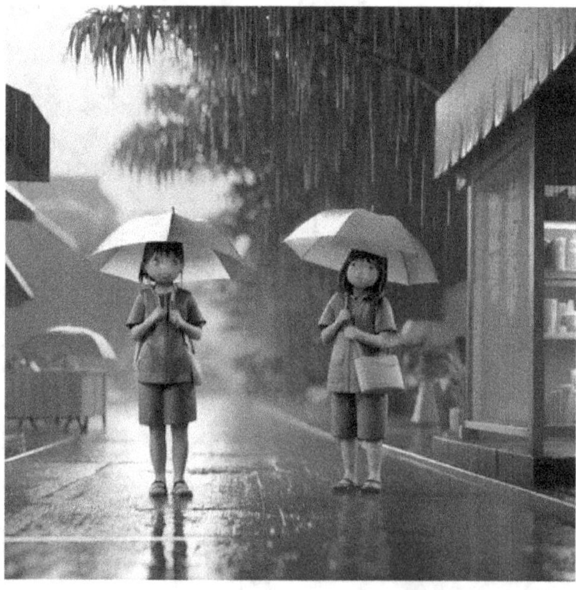

How To Stay Healthy In Winter Season

Remaining healthy throughout the winter time of year can be trying because of colder temperatures, shorter days, and the pervasiveness of colds and influenza.

Below are thirty ways to keep your health in check during the winter months:

Nutrition

1. Eat Produce in Season: Include root vegetables, kale, Brussels sprouts, and other winter vegetables in your meals.

2. Remain Hydrated: Drink a lot of water, natural teas, and stocks to remain hydrated, regardless of whether you feel as parched.

3. To support your immune system, include foods high in zinc (nuts, seeds) and vitamin C (citrus fruits, bell peppers).

4. Limit Sugar Consumption: Avoid sugary snacks and beverages because they can weaken your immune system.

5. Cook Warm Feasts: Plan generous soups and stews that are nutritious and warming.

6. Nibble Shrewdly: Pick healthy bites like nuts, yogurt, or natural products rather than packed snacks.

7. Think about Enhancements: Converse with a medical care supplier about vitamin D enhancements, particularly on the off chance that you have restricted sun openness.

Actual work

8. Remain Dynamic Inside: Take part in indoor activities like yoga, pilates, or home exercise recordings.

9. Wrap Up for Outside Exercises: Take strolls, climbs, or runs while dressed properly for the climate.

10. Join an Exercise center or Class: Consider joining a nearby rec center or wellness class to remain persuaded and dynamic.

11. Try Winter Sports: For fun exercise, try winter sports like skiing, snowboarding, or ice skating.

 12. Set an Everyday practice: Timetable customary exercise times to keep yourself responsible.

Mental Wellness

13. Get Sunlight: You can improve your mood and vitamin D levels by going outside during the day.

14. Practice Care: Take part in care or reflection to lessen pressure and work on mental prosperity.

 15. Maintain Social Connections: Calls, video chats, and safe in-person gatherings are all ways to maintain social connections.

16. Reduce the amount of time spent in front of a screen to avoid feeling isolated and anxious.

17. Hobbies: Engage in activities that bring you joy and fulfillment during your spare time.

Sleep

18. Keep a Rest Timetable: Hit the hay and wake up simultaneously every day to control your rest cycle.

19. Establish a Comfortable Rest Climate: Keep your room dim, calm, and at an agreeable temperature.

20. Reduce your intake of stimulants and depressants, especially in the evening, and drink less alcohol.

Health and hygiene practices

21. Wash your hands frequently to stop the spread of germs and practice good hand hygiene.

22. Get Vaccinated: You should think about getting the flu shot and any other vaccines that are recommended

. 23. Remain at Home When Debilitated: Assuming you feel unwell, set aside some margin to rest and recuperate to forestall spreading sickness.

24. Utilize a Humidifier: Keep indoor air sodden to assist with forestalling dry skin and respiratory issues.

Beauty Tips

25. Use a good moisturizer on a regular basis to combat the dry skin brought on by the cold weather.

26. Protect Your Skin: On sunny winter days, especially if you go skiing or spend time outside, put on sunscreen.

General Prosperity

27. Keep a gratitude journal to focus on the good things in your life and practice gratitude.

28. Put forth Reasonable Objectives: Put forth feasible wellbeing and health objectives for the colder time of year.

29. Reduce holiday stress by planning ahead for holiday events to avoid stress at the last minute.

30. If you're having problems with your mental health, don't be afraid to talk to a professional. You can help maintain your mental and physical health during the colder months by incorporating these suggestions into your winter routine.

How To Stay Healthy In Summer Season

As the late spring sun blasts down, it tends to be trying to remain cool and agreeable. High temperatures can prompt distress, drying out, and even intensity related illnesses. In any case, with a couple of shrewd procedures, you can partake in the late spring while at the same time keeping the intensity under control. The following are some tips to assist you with beating the intensity this mid year season.

1. Remain Hydrated: Drink a lot of water over the course of the day. Aim for at least eight glasses per day, and if you exercise or spend time outside, drink more.

2. Wear a light outfit. Settle on baggy, light-hued clothing produced using breathable textures like cotton or material. Your body will stay cooler as a result.

3. Apply sunscreen. To shield your skin from harmful UV rays, use a broad-spectrum sunscreen with at least SPF 30. Especially after swimming or sweating, reapply every two hours.

4. Shade Search :Stay in shade whenever possible, especially between 10 a.m. and 4 p.m., when the sun is at its strongest. This can altogether diminish your openness to coordinate daylight.

5. Shower in cool water. You can get instant relief from the heat by taking a cool shower or bath to lower your body temperature.

6. Use Fans Carefully :Roof fans and convenient fans can assist with flowing air. For a cooling effect, position fans so that they blow air directly over you.

7. Close the blinds and curtains. Reduce indoor temperatures by closing curtains and blinds during the hottest parts of the day to block out sunlight.

8. Eat Little Foods :Eat fruits and salads, which are lighter and easier to digest. Eat light, hot meals sparingly, as these can raise your body temperature.

9. Remain Inside During Pinnacle Intensity :During the hottest parts of the day, avoid going out in the sun. When the weather is cooler, schedule your excursions for early in the morning or late at night.

10. Employ a Cool Cloth. To help you cool down quickly, dampen a cloth with cold water and place it on your forehead, neck, or wrists.

11.Buy air conditioning. To keep your home cool, use air conditioning whenever possible. If you don't have air conditioning, you might want to go to malls.

12. Make Your Own Air Conditioner. Place a bowl of ice in front of a fan and fill it with ice. The air will blow over the ice, making a cool wind.

13. Remain Dynamic :
In the first part of the day In the event that you work out, do it in the early morning when temperatures are cooler. You won't get too hot from this.

14. Use Cooling Gel Items: Consider utilizing cooling gels or salves that can give a reviving sensation on your skin.

 15. Hydrate with Organic products :Consolidate hydrating natural products like watermelon, cucumbers, and oranges into your eating regimen. Not only are they cooling, but they're also full of water.

16. Keep away from Caffeine and Liquor :Alcohol and caffeine can dehydrate you. Instead, choose herbal teas or water.

 17. Take pauses :Take frequent breaks in the shade or inside if you're working or exercising outside to cool down.

 18. Spray water with it. Convey a little shower bottle loaded up with water and fog your face and body to chill over the course of the day.

19. Cool Your House. Use heat-intelligent window movies or shades to keep your home cooler. The temperature inside can be significantly reduced by this.

20. Make plans for water sports: To keep cool, try water-based activities like kayaking, swimming, or just splashing around in a pool.

21. Use a damp cloth. To assist in cooling down, wrap a damp towel around your wrists or neck.

22. Avoid strenuous endeavors. Avoid doing anything strenuous during the hottest parts of the day. Settle on lighter undertakings that will not overheat you.

23. Stay up to date Keep an eye on heat advisories and weather forecasts. You can better plan your activities if you are informed.

24. Utilize Regular Ventilation :Open windows during cooler nights to allow in natural air, and close them during the day to keep the intensity out.

25. Make Your Sleeping Space Cool: Utilize lightweight sheet material and save your room dim and cool for a superior night's rest.

26. Stay in touch. Verify how friends and family, particularly the elderly, are coping with the heat.

27. Apply ice packs. To quickly cool down, apply ice packs to pulse points like your wrists, neck, and ankles.

28. Plan Indoor Exercises :To keep cool while having fun, plan indoor activities like movie nights or board games.

29. Pay attention to Your Body :Pay close attention to symptoms of heat exhaustion like nausea, dizziness, or excessive sweating. Assuming that you experience these side effects, look for shade, hydrate, and cool down right away.

30. Avoid spicy foods in the summer season.

31. Wear light cotton clothes.

Liver and Pancreas

The liver and pancreas are essential organs that assume vital parts in keeping up with generally speaking wellbeing. The liver is answerable for detoxifying hurtful substances, creating bile for absorption, and directing digestion. It likewise stores fundamental supplements and nutrients. In contrast, the pancreas is responsible for the production of hormones that control blood sugar levels, such as insulin, as well as digestive enzymes. These organs work together to maintain metabolic equilibrium, digestion, and nutrient absorption, highlighting their significance for disease prevention and wellness. Keeping up with their wellbeing is fundamental for a flourishing body. Dealing with your pancreas is critical for keeping up with in general wellbeing and forestalling different illnesses. Nine things you can do to keep your pancreas healthy:

1. Reduce weight: over weight is a risk factor for pancreatitis and pancreatic disease. By keeping a healthy weight through a reasonable eating routine and standard activity, you can diminish your risk of pancreatic issues.

2. Eat a decent eating regimen: Consume an eating routine wealthy in natural products, vegetables, entire grains, lean proteins, and sound fats. Limit your admission of handled food varieties, immersed fats, and sugars, which can add to pancreatic issues.

3. Limit alcohol consumption: Pancreatitis, a painful and potentially dangerous condition, can result from excessive alcohol consumption. Limit your liquor admission to advance a healthy pancreas.

4. Stop smoking: Smoking is a critical risk factor for pancreatic malignant growth. Assuming you smoke, stopping can incredibly decrease your risk of fostering this lethal infection and assist with keeping up with your pancreas wellbeing.

5. Remain hydrated: Drinking a sufficient amount of water is significant for general wellbeing, including your pancreas. Appropriate hydration assists your pancreas with working ideally.

6. Limit your sugar intake: Consuming a lot of sugar can make you overweight or have type 2 diabetes, both of which can put pressure on the pancreas. Keep your pancreas healthy by avoiding sugary foods and beverages.

7. Stress or Depression: Persistent stress can adversely influence your wellbeing, including your pancreas. Practice pressure diminishing exercises like meditate, profound breathing, yoga, or leisure activities you appreciate to hold your feelings of anxiety under control.

8. Get customary check-ups: Normal visits to your medical services supplier can assist with distinguishing any potential pancreatic issues from the beginning. Examine your risk factors and any worries you have about your pancreas during these visits.

9. Know your family ancestry: A few pancreatic problems, as genetic pancreatitis, can run in families. You and your healthcare provider can assess your risk and, if necessary, take preventative measures with the assistance of an understanding of your family history.

Keep in mind, keeping a solid way of life is vital to supporting your pancreas and in general prosperity. In the event that you have any worries about your pancreas or generally wellbeing, counsel your medical services supplier for customized exhortation and direction.

Keeping a healthy liver is significant for generally speaking prosperity as the liver assumes a fundamental part in detoxification, digestion, and different other fundamental capabilities in the body.

The following are few tips to assist with keeping your liver sound:

1. Maintain weight: obesity can expand the risk of fatty liver infection and other liver issues. Maintain weight through a reasonable eating routine and normal activity.

2. Eat a reasonable eating regimen: Consume a lot of natural products, vegetables, entire grains, lean proteins, and healthy fats to help liver wellbeing

3. Limit liquor utilization: Inordinate liquor admission can prompt liver harm. On the off chance that you drink, do as such with some restraint or consider taking out liquor.

4. Remain hydrated: Hydrate everyday to assist with flushing poisons from your body and backing liver capability.

5. Limit processed food varieties: processed food varieties can be high in unhealthy fats, added substances, and sugars that can strain the liver. Select entire, normal food varieties whenever the situation allows

. 6. Limit sugar consumption: High sugar admission can add to fatty liver illness. Lessen your utilization of sweet food varieties and drinks.

7. Maintain a healthy cholesterol level because elevated levels can result in fatty liver deposits. Hold your cholesterol under control through a sound eating routine and normal activity.

8. Work-out routinely: Active work can assist with diminishing liver fat, further develop digestion, and advance in general wellbeing.

9. Oversee pressure: Persistent pressure can affect liver capability. Engage in stress-relieving activities like yoga, deep breathing, or meditation.

 10. Get immunization: Inoculation against hepatitis A and B can assist with forestalling liver diseases that can cause long term harm.

11. Try not to share individual things: Hepatitis infections can spread through the sharing of individual things like razors or toothbrushes. To reduce the likelihood of infection, don't share such items.

 12. Practice safe sex: Hepatitis infections can likewise be sent physically. To stop the spread of infections, have safe sex.

13. Limit exposure to toxins: Avoid exposing yourself to chemicals and pollutants in the environment, which can harm the liver. Utilize defensive gear while working with harmful substances.

14. Stay away from unlawful medications: Unlawful medications can seriously harm the liver. To safeguard liver health, refrain from using illegal substances.

15. Adhere to medicine directions: follw prescriptions as recommended by your medical services supplier.

Some Disease associated with liver and Pancreas that can be prevent or control by following above tips:

1. Hepatitis: This is when the liver gets inflamed, usually from viruses like A, B, C, D, and E, too much alcohol, or autoimmune issues. Signs include feeling tired, yellow skin and eyes, stomach pain, and dark urine.

2. Fatty Liver Disease: This happens when too much fat builds up in the liver, either from drinking too much alcohol (alcoholic fatty liver) or being overweight, having diabetes, or metabolic issues (non-alcoholic fatty liver). Early signs might not show up, but it can lead to liver damage or scarring.

3. Cirrhosis: This is a serious condition where the liver gets scarred and can't work properly, often from long-term liver diseases or alcohol abuse. Symptoms include feeling tired, bruising easily, swelling in the legs and belly, and confusion.

Pancreas Issues

1. Pancreatitis: This is when the pancreas gets inflamed, which can be short-term or long-term. Short-term pancreatitis is usually from gallstones or drinking too much. Long-term pancreatitis can happen after short-term episodes. Symptoms include severe stomach pain, feeling sick to your stomach, throwing up, and fever.

2. Diabetes Mellitus: This is when the pancreas can't make enough insulin (Type 1) or the body doesn't use it well (Type 2). It can cause high blood sugar, leading to heart problems, kidney damage, and nerve damage.

3. Pancreatic Cancer: This is a type of cancer that starts in the pancreas and is often found late because the symptoms are vague. Risk factors include smoking, being overweight, and having a family history of pancreatic cancer. Symptoms might include losing weight, yellow skin, and stomach pain.

4. Exocrine Pancreatic Insufficiency (EPI): This is when the pancreas doesn't make enough digestive enzymes, causing problems with absorbing nutrients. Symptoms include losing weight, diarrhea, and having fatty stools. EPI can be caused by long-term pancreatitis, cystic fibrosis, or pancreatic cancer.

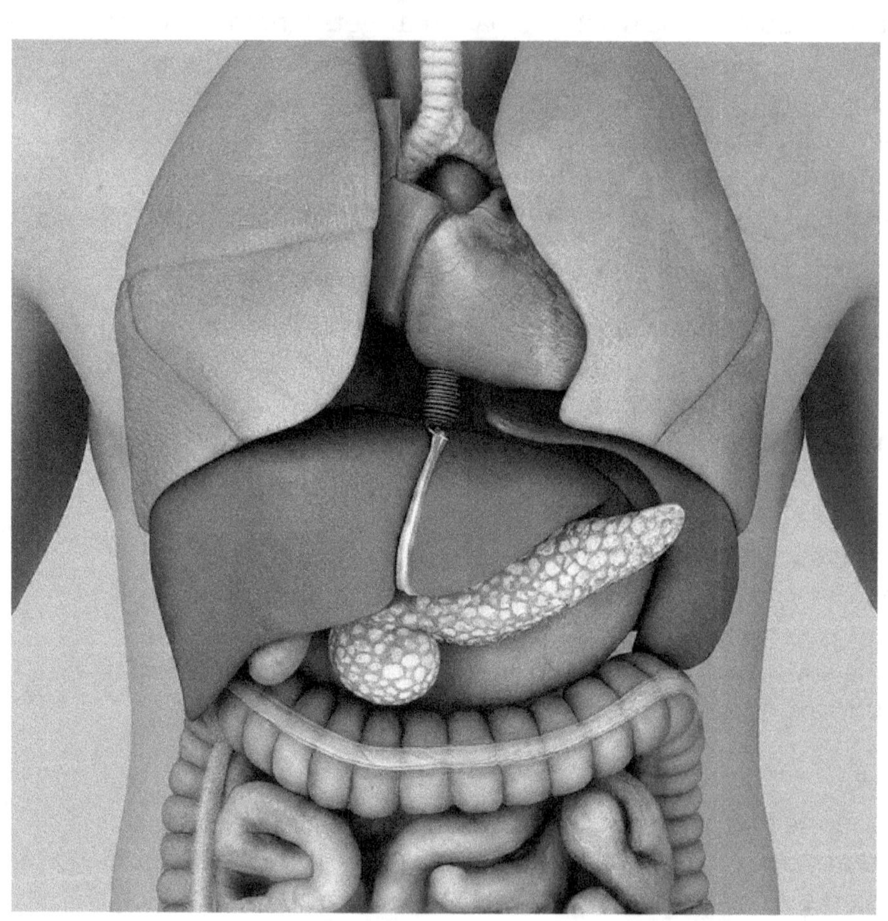

Congratulations on reaching the final page of this book! Your journey towards a healthier and happier life has just begun. Remember, wellness is not a destination but a continuous effort to nourish your mind, body, and soul. Here are some key takeaways to carry forward:

1. Prioritize Self-Care: Make time for yourself every day. Whether it's a moment of mindfulness, a walk in nature, or indulging in a hobby, self-care is crucial for your overall well-being.

2. Embrace Balance: Strive for balance in all aspects of your life – from your diet and exercise routine to your work and relationships. Moderation is key to sustainable health.

3. Stay Informed: Stay curious and keep learning about health and wellness. The more you know, the better equipped you are to make informed choices that benefit your health.

4. Listen to Your Body: Your body is unique, and it often communicates its needs clearly. Pay attention to how you feel and respond accordingly. Rest when you need to, move when you can, and nourish yourself with wholesome foods.

5. Build a Support System: Surround yourself with people who uplift and support your health goals. Share your journey with loved ones and seek help when needed. Remember, you're not alone in this pursuit of wellness.

As you close this book, remember that every small step you take towards a healthier lifestyle matters. Celebrate your achievements, learn from setbacks, and keep moving forward. Your health is your most valuable asset – cherish it, nurture it, and watch it flourish.

Thank you for embarking on this journey with us. We wish you a life filled with vibrant health, endless energy, and boundless joy.

Here's to your well-being and a future
brimming with possibilities!

With best wishes,

Hajra Begum

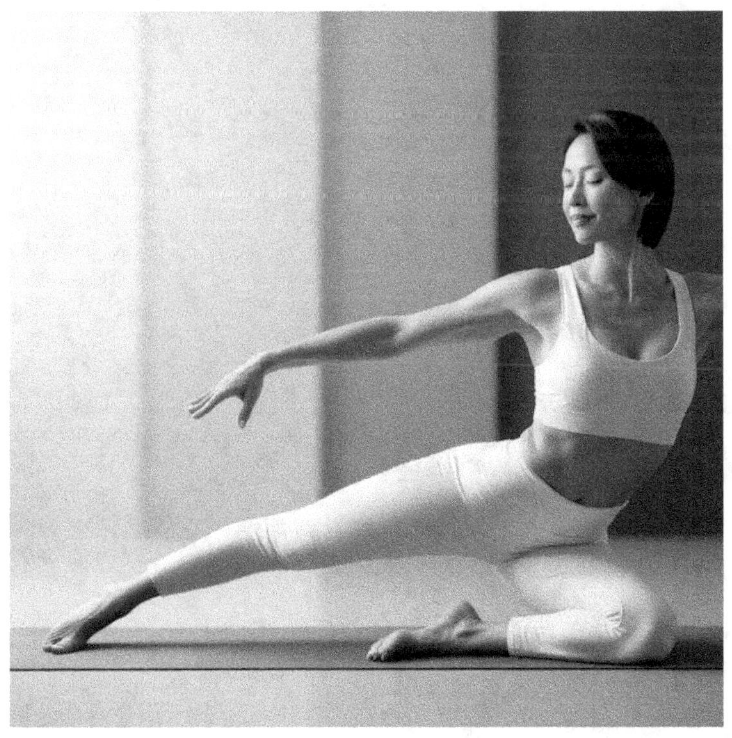